80 YEARS WITHOUT DEMENTIA

Diagnosis *Doesn't* Define Life

Lisa Twigg

First published in 2023 by LisaTwigg

© LisaTwigg
The moral rights of the author have been asserted.
This book is an Inspirational Book Writers book.

Author:

Twigg, Lisa

Title:

80 Years Without Dementia; Diagnosis *Doesn't* Define Life

ISBN:

9798857650264

Editor-in-chief: Keziah Daniel
Cover Design: Sarah Rose Graphic Design

Disclaimer:
The material in this publication is of the nature of general professional advice, but it is not intended to provide specific guidance for particular circumstances and it should not be relied on as the basis for any decision to take action or not take action on any particular matter which it covers. Readers should obtain individual advice from the author where appropriate, before making any such decision. To the maximum extent permitted by law, the author and publisher disclaim all responsibility and liability to any person, arising directly or indirectly from any person taking or not taking action based on the information in this publication.

DEDICATION

This book is dedicated to my dad, Bob.

He's half the reason I made it onto the planet in the first place, and he's taught me many things as I've gone through childhood, teenagerhood, adulthood, and parenthood. The lessons he has taught our family in the final years of his life were the impetus for this book, and I'm both honoured and proud to bring them to you.

I've always loved you Dad, and I always will.

PRAISE FOR 80 YEARS WITHOUT DEMENTIA

Lisa's book '80 Years Without Dementia' is a wonderful tribute to her father, Bob. It provides an insight into Bob's life as a loving husband, father and a valued member of the community. The story then takes the reader on an emotional journey through Bob's diagnosis of dementia at 81 and the impact this had on Bob, his wife and family. Lisa talks about the difficult and heartbreaking decision they had to make when the time came for Bob to go into care. It is an inspiring story that talks about the difficulties faced when someone has dementia, but Lisa has also been able to find the positives in a sad situation and beautifully describes the things she is grateful for. The quotes at the beginning of the chapters and 'take home message' at the end of each one is a bonus for the reader. Lisa has included a chapter on 'Help and Support' which is a valuable resource for anyone faced with a similar situation. Lisa's words 'it's not all bad all of the time' can be a source of hope for anyone confronted with a difficult life situation.

Kathy Carpenter, Accredited Mental Health Social Worker

This book offers heartfelt insights to support loved ones with dementia. It's full of heart and vulnerability, delivering contextual information that is immensely supportive. I believe this will bring emotional release, understanding, and healing to readers. Very well done on a beautiful book that WILL touch hearts and change lives for the better.

Keziah Daniel, Editor

FOREWORD

Living with dementia is challenging, it's a slow goodbye to one's memories and independence, and it brings irreversible changes to relationships and lifestyle. According to ABS data, it is sadly now the second most common cause of death in Australia. Whilst so much is being done to promote early diagnosis and treatment, there is still no cure.

Capturing the nuanced changes that occur is what Lisa has done beautifully in her book. A dementia diagnosis does not define someone, but it definitely does teach us valuable lessons for those willing to lean in. Lisa has leaned in deeply, as a daughter, as a social worker, as a community leader, to share her family's experience of dementia uncut, raw, and vulnerably.

I first met Lisa in 2021 on the phone, enquiring about the Moreton Bay Dementia Alliance and exploring how she wanted to find meaning for her father's dementia through research participation, the arts or volunteer projects. I was impressed by her willingness to embrace dementia and her desire to turn pain into gain, to pave the way for others. We discussed various potential opportunities which has led her to write this poignant legacy for her Dad.

Everyone's lived experience of dementia is unique and different, however some stages and behaviours are similar. The feelings of fear, frustration, guilt, and grief expressed will no doubt resonate for many, and hopefully by reading this book move you to a place of acceptance and gratitude.

80 Years Without Dementia is an inspiring, emotive memoir, a highly readable personal account of how dementia has been a gift, rather than a curse to Lisa's family. It has practical take home messages, powerful curated insights and should be read with an open heart by all who have a loved one living with dementia and by all committed to creating dementia friendly communities around our nation and globe.

Kerri - Anne Dooley, RN

Managing Director, My Care Enterprises
Co-Founder and Chair, Moreton Bay Dementia Alliance

TABLE OF CONTENTS

INTRODUCTION

This book is a legacy for my dad

It is the parting gift he is unable to deliver himself, but for which I am the conduit. **Via the teaching of valuable life lessons, this book is his way of reframing dementia and giving back to the community one last time.** Let me explain.

A glimpse into the inspiring life of my dad

Dad has always been a very community-minded person and was involved with various committees, projects, and organisations at a local level. He was a Bushfire Captain in our farming district for many years, proud that he never let a fire get away on his watch! Back in the '60s, he was instrumental in getting the telephone connected in our area (prior to that, communication was via the Royal Flying Doctor Service radio); Dad was part of the committee who successfully established a kindergarten in our local town; He was heavily involved in Landcare Australia, for which he was awarded Citizen of the Year in 1989, and nominated for the 'Peoplescape' installation at Parliament House in 2001; My dad played in the local basketball competition well into his thirties; He was an Elder in the local Presbyterian Church...........

You get the idea. Community was important to Dad, and the idea of "doing your bit" and being generous with your time is an attitude he has passed on to my brothers and me as we have grown up.

Dad was an intelligent man, had a very enquiring mind, and was driven to get the best out of himself. In his forties, he enrolled, as an external student, in university for the first time and completed a number of courses. When my eldest brother went away to boarding school, Dad studied for his private pilot's licence, so it would be quicker and easier to come and go to the farm (75 minutes one-way instead of 5 hours by road), not only for us away at school, but also for getting parts and equipment when farm machinery broke down or needed repair. And after back surgery aged fifty, he was told the best thing for him would be to swim as much as possible – Dad was not a swimmer and, at that time, the closest pool was 180km away! But being the focused (some would say stubborn!) man that he was, he took lessons, prioritised the need to swim regularly, and set about getting to a pool whenever and wherever he could, something he continued to do even into his eighties.

What's my intention in writing this book?

So, what's all this got to do with life lessons and dementia? Fair question. For quite a while now, I have felt an overwhelming need to bring Dad's experience with dementia to life, but in a way that attempts to reframe (at least part of) the journey from a negative into a positive. **The drive has come from my desire to write something heartfelt, which may help reduce fear for others, provide hope that 'it's not all bad all of the time', reduce the stigma around dementia, and give some insight into what might come up along the way, particularly in relation to emotions.**

What's the big idea for the book?

You read above that I refer to this legacy for my dad as his 'parting gift' to the community, but I will take it further than that and suggest dementia has actually been a gift to our family – one we have only received in the last years of Dad's life. I know that may sound controversial, and you may be thinking it also sounds callous, uncaring, heartless, and disrespectful to him. But I don't see it that way, and I'm very confident he wouldn't either. **The reason I see it as a gift, and that's ultimately what has driven me to write this book, is that I believe there are life lessons to be learned when you open your** mind to the fact that 'everything happens for a reason' and there is always a positive tucked away somewhere.

Dad has always been an optimist, a 'glass-half-full' kind of guy. If you went to him hoping to wallow in self-pity or get his support on why your situation was terribly bad, you would probably leave empty-handed! He was always the antidote to negativity – whenever he was challenged by situations in his life, he maintained an ability to identify the positives, or at the very least not dwell on the negatives. He has instilled in us, myself and my two brothers, the need to consider things from a glass-half-full point of view. And I think that's why I view Dad's dementia as having provided us with a gift. It has forced us to think about the life lessons we have learned (and are still learning) as we've gone through this journey with him, those lessons being everything from slowing down to appreciate the simple things in life, to being courageous when hard decisions must be made.

If even one person could take something from this book or benefit from learning about someone else's experience with dementia, Dad would see that very much as a positive. "A gift that keeps on giving", so to speak, even after his own life comes to an end and he is no longer able to teach in person.

What are the basics of our family story?

In the two and a half years leading up to his dementia diagnosis, Dad was assessed twice by a neurologist and told he had stress-induced short-term memory loss. What prompted those visits to neurology was the subtle changes we had been noticing (over a period of 5 or 6 years) in Dad's capacity. He was then diagnosed with dementia at the beginning of 2018, at the age of 81 (hence the title of the book 😊). Mum and Dad have lived at home with my family and me (in a granny flat under our house) since the end of 2012, though Dad moved into residential care in 2021. His facility is little more than a five-minute drive from our house, relatively close to the beach. We consider ourselves very blessed to have found him a suitable place to live so close to home.

Where are we at now?

At the time of writing, Dad is 86 years old, soon to be 87. Right now, Dad can still eat (albeit not as much and very slowly), he can still walk (slowly and with a walking frame), he can still talk (though not always coherently these days), and he can still enjoy going out with us or coming home for a few hours. He is in decline and will likely reach a stage where all those things will be compromised, and some of the physical challenges will be more intense. I know there may also come a time when he won't know our faces anymore, and we won't be able to bring joy into his day in the same way we can now. My mission for that time is to embrace the lessons we have learned through this journey (which will unfold for you in the upcoming pages), be in the moment with him, and love him as much as possible. Dad doesn't want to linger in a 'vegetative' state at the end of his life, he's always said that, but unfortunately our laws won't allow us to relieve him of his suffering when we feel he's reached a point where the disease has completely overtaken him. Thankfully, we are not there yet, but if or when we are, we will have no choice but to draw on all the wonderful memories we have of Dad and celebrate the full and happy life he has lived.

What is dementia?

So now you know a bit about our story. What you may not know is what dementia is, so allow me to give you a quick definition before we go any further. Dementia is an umbrella term for several diseases that affect memory, thinking, and the ability to perform daily activities. You may be familiar with the most common disease, Alzheimer's, but there are also Vascular, Lewy body, Frontotemporal, and a few other types of dementia. Initially Dad was thought to have Vascular Dementia (having had blood pressure issues for many years), but it was later suggested it might be Alzheimer's, or possibly a mix from more than one cause.

What to expect from this book?

The layout of this book is such that each chapter focuses on a particular topic, basically each of the lessons Dad's dementia has taught us (and in some cases, is still teaching us). Most of the content is delivered as a narrative, though there are some places where point form was used if that best suited the issue being discussed. At the end of each chapter, there is a 'take-home message', and most chapters open with a quote that conveys the essence of the upcoming insights. My hope is that you will be inspired by the insights we've gained through our experience and use them to support you in your own life, whether dementia is part of your story or not.

Okay, let's jump straight into the first chapter, and you'll hear quite a bit from Mum. If you're unfamiliar with dementia, this will give you insight into some of the challenges and emotions this disease throws up on an ongoing basis. If you're living with dementia, close to someone who is, or working in the field, I'm sure you'll find some of what she talks about resonates with you and makes a whole lot of sense.

I hope you enjoy reading the book, it is an honour for me to write it on behalf of my beloved Mum and Dad.

CHAPTER ONE

THE (PARALLEL) EMOTIONAL JOURNEY OF THE CARER

This chapter is largely about Mum, though you'll also hear a bit about Dad at the beginning. Mum and Dad have been married for sixty-two years at the time of writing, and Mum was Dad's primary carer for three and a half years post-diagnosis (and as I said in the Introduction, his cognitive capacity had been declining for several years before that). Since Dad has been in residential care, Mum has visited him or taken him out four or five times most weeks. After the 'Partners in Care' initiative was introduced into his facility, she was permitted to visit Dad during COVID lockdowns, but only under the proviso that she wore a gown, an N95 mask, and latex gloves. She is, therefore, well-qualified to be the focus of this chapter! I ask you to respect the vulnerability she has shown in the sharing of her words. I am so proud of her honesty in helping me paint a picture of what can be a very challenging and confronting world. The world of dementia.

The (parallel) journey of the full-time primary carer is emotional, and it is also very hard at times. I could probably have filled a book just recounting, from Mum's perspective, some of the many experiences she has had and all the emotions she has felt as we've gone down the dementia path with Dad, particularly in the years he was living at home. But there are other parts of that journey I want to introduce too, so I'm going to give you a brief snapshot of some of the behaviours Dad has exhibited as his dementia has progressed. I will also give you a glimpse into some of the emotions which have come up (some of it with direct quotes from Mum in *italics*). If you are not familiar with dementia, I hope this helps set the scene from the carer's point of view.

If you do already have some familiarity with dementia, I'm sure you will recognise some of what I've written, and it may resonate with you in quite a profound way.

Maybe it seems obvious, but it's probably important to point out at this stage that each person presents with dementia in their own individual way. Though there may be similarities to the ways in which others present, their behaviours differ, the rate of their decline is varied, their needs are unique to them, and their persona is their own. Similarly, everyone caring for someone living with dementia is different, they experience the challenges in their own way, and they bring their individual coping threshold to that role.

Some of the challenging behaviours Dad exhibited as time went on were as follows:

- Ongoing night-time disturbance – regularly waking Mum up, shining a torch in her face, getting up and dressed in the middle of the night, turning on all the lights, preparing something to eat, and so on

- 'Shadowing' Mum around the flat

- Repeatedly asking the same questions, making the same statements, and requesting the same things

- Changing his clothes throughout the day

- Moving things around, making and remaking the bed many times over, reorganising bits and pieces

- Non-believing or rejecting information, often becoming argumentative

- Restlessness, unable to settle with a task or activity, losing interest in previous hobbies and pastimes

- Deteriorating ability to help, but always wanting to try (lawn mowing, pruning, raking, cutting up vegetables, sorting washing) and therefore requiring increased supervision

- Wandering away from the agreed waiting spot, maybe in front of the shop or at a table in a café

Whilst Dad has presented as scared or fearful on some occasions, seemingly confused by his own thoughts (which at times have appeared hallucinatory), we are grateful for the fact he has not become highly aggressive or violent as some others do. There was an occasion when an undiagnosed infection led to him grabbing a staff member in his residential facility, as she was trying to stop him from doing something, and in another instance, he retaliated after another resident took a swipe at him. But, overall, his behaviours have been very consistent with his declining cognitive state, and we have always tried to keep reevaluating them through the lens of it being the disease which makes things challenging, not Dad himself.

Now let's take a glimpse into some of the emotions which have come up along the way

Shock – A formal dementia diagnosis was quite a long time coming for Dad. For several years in the lead-up to the first neurology appointment in 2015, and before the follow-up consult twelve months later, we had been noticing significant changes in his capacity, and he was very aware his memory was not razor sharp as it had been previously. He was greatly relieved when he was told, at both those neurology appointments, that he did not have dementia, because he'd heard enough to know dementia wouldn't be something he wanted. I still remember him and Mum coming home from the first appointment and Dad announcing, quite choked up, "Well, it's not THE BIG D word, so that's good". He was happy, very happy in fact; short-term memory loss was something he was prepared to accept. He bought a book about brain neuroplasticity and was quite optimistic about 'retraining his brain' to restore some of its previous cognitive function.

However, as the decline continued, and it was obvious short-term memory loss was NOT the only issue we were dealing with (we were seeing poor judgement, lack of focus, inability to plan, and so on), we pushed for further testing. And the dementia diagnosis finally came from the local memory clinic at the beginning of 2018. Despite the long lead-up time, it did deliver a shock to both Mum and Dad, I guess because it finalised what had been quite a long and drawn-out process. Dad now has dementia – what does that mean? What do we do next? What can we still do before he gets any worse? How long will he live? What help is there? Do we need to buy anything in particular? Are there any treatment options? You get the idea.

Denial – Following close on the heels of the shock came some denial, more from Dad than Mum. To be honest, I think his ability to take on the diagnosis was already a bit limited by that time, and thankfully, I think he had also lost the fear that was previously there about dementia, so it wasn't something that caused him ongoing worry. He would still have periods of relative clarity where he knew something wasn't quite right, but he couldn't necessarily articulate what the problem was. He'd say, "Ugh, I used to know this sort of thing, but my memory is not what it used to be", though he wasn't necessarily aware he had dementia. In fact, sometimes when Mum would tell him, in an attempt to explain a situation to him, he'd look at her with raised eyebrows as if to say, "What, me?" Mum does recall one conversation when she told Dad he had been diagnosed with dementia, and he crossed his arms and said, "I don't like it" though he didn't dwell on it, probably because the moment passed and he moved on.

Immediately after Dad was diagnosed, his GP told him straight up he would need to hand in his driver's license (something we had been encouraging him to do for a while), and that became the main message he took from that appointment. He became intent on trying to get his license reinstated for a while afterwards, as he was under the (false) impression he'd been asked to hand it in due to his age, not for any other reason. He got quite annoyed about it several times and even walked up to the Department of Transport to enquire about it at one stage. Thankfully this pursuit died a natural death with a bit of time, and he gave up questioning where their big four-wheel-drive had gone or why Mum always insisted on driving (now in a compact little Toyota!!)

Grief (ongoing) – Mum didn't linger in denial for very long. She was more able to accept a diagnosis as she had known something was wrong for quite a long period of time and, like me, had worked out it was more than just short-term memory loss. For her, grief and what was going to be lost were the more significant emotions which followed diagnosis:

> *"The grief, it didn't stop, it was sort of continuing because I didn't know what was going to happen, and I felt really sad for Dad. I was grieving for what he was going to be losing and what we were going to be losing. And a lot of it was really unknown stuff – though I'd heard so much about people with dementia, and I had a fairly good idea that it wasn't going to be something easy. And the grief is probably still ongoing...each time things happen or when I go to visit Dad sometimes......when I can see him declining and, you know, he can't speak properly, and I wonder whether he knows who I am, that sort of thing. I often come away with grief... it's grief for what you've lost"*.

Loss (ongoing) – Mum turned 81 a few months after Dad went into residential care, and at that time his facility was in lockdown, meaning we were unable to visit or bring him out for the day. This was the first time he had ever missed a birthday with Mum, and she felt it keenly. Other simple examples of how the sense of loss is ongoing include suddenly cooking for one instead of two, the fact that Dad has been unable to fully comprehend Mother's Day, Christmas, Father's Day, or his own birthday for quite some time now, and going out for dinner less often (because it's not much fun on your own). There are also the physical losses. It's not that Dad doesn't welcome Mum holding his hand or giving him a hug anymore; he simply wouldn't think of it and can't initiate it himself. At some point when Dad's night-time waking reached crisis point, we made the decision to put a bed for Mum into their open-plan living area, hoping this might help (which it didn't) cut down his overnight disturbances. Reflecting on that time, Mum spoke of how it felt when she could no longer sleep next to the person she'd been sleeping with for six decades, just like she no longer had a partner with whom she could talk through feelings, ideas, family matters, or health issues as she had always done.

In relation to his grandkids, Mum commented:

> *"There are lots of times when he's here, the grandkids are here, and we're chatting, and you can see he's not really tuning into what's going on. That's the loss, the loss for him, and that makes it sad."*

It does make it sad; however, I think I can say with confidence that the sense of loss we feel is more acute for us than it is for Dad, at least at this late stage in his journey. There's no doubt he experienced a sense of both grief and loss as his capabilities and memory were starting to be negatively impacted, though I suspect these feelings had already been overtaken by his decline around the time his diagnosis was formalised. There's a chapter a bit further on about "living in the moment", and I guess this is what delivers us comfort – knowing Dad is living in the moment and (seemingly) not consumed by an ongoing sense of grief.

Anger – Mum did experience anger at the time of Dad's diagnosis, but that faded relatively quickly as she reached the point of acceptance. As you can probably imagine though, having read through some of the challenging behaviours dementia throws up, there were many times Mum felt, and expressed, anger towards Dad. She was constantly sleep-deprived, had very few in-home or external support hours (Dad was on a low-level care package), and was over eighty herself by the time Dad went into care. As you will read in the next chapter, I pretty much "called time" on Dad living at home, but I recently asked Mum if she had ever got to the point in her own head where she was so angry with Dad that she thought she couldn't care for him anymore:

"There were a few times I actually said to him I can't do this anymore, it's getting too hard....I'm too tired. I'm gonna have to do something different. I'm gonna have to put you somewhere to be looked after. And then after that I'd think ah, that was a terrible thing to say. I certainly don't want to do that. But I certainly thought that in my head a number of times, especially when I was really shouting and yelling and then so tired and I couldn't sleep. All that sort of thing....almost like an empty threat... There were certainly times when I thought, Oh my god, who is this person? I don't even like this person, going on like that and look at me, I'm all stressed. And then, when I'd calm down, I'd quite often just go up and give Dad a hug...I'd know it's not his fault".

Fear (of the unknown) – Not only the unknowns around how quickly the disease might progress, how it would manifest itself for Dad, or how long he has left, but it was quite daunting for Mum when the decline of her previously highly capable life partner meant they had to switch roles and she had to start taking on, for the first time in her late 70's, the tasks he had always done in their marriage – paying bills, comparing insurance, doing the banking, getting the car serviced, etc. Whilst we were able to help her navigate through those things, it was unsettling and something she had never planned for at a time when there were so many other uncertainties.

Emotional exhaustion – As you have already heard, Mum became more and more exhausted as Dad's cognitive function declined over time, and a large part of that was due to ongoing night-time disturbance:

"I can remember a number of times at night, you know he'd be in and out with the torch, I would be so frustrated, I'd absolutely bounce out of bed and say, "Put that torch down, what are you

doing?" I'd be grabbing the torch off him....and he'd be holding it, we'd be juggling with the torch.......so you know, those sorts of things, it was just a reaction. I mean, I'd never talk like that normally or do that, but there were a number of those sorts of things where you just cannot tolerate any more. It'd be like, here he comes again with the bloody thing shining it everywhere. Certainly there was a lot of guilt after those episodes."

Along with a lack of quality sleep, Mum's exhaustion also stemmed from the fact it was a bit like having a toddler all over again, in some respects – the requirement for constant supervision, being followed everywhere, having to redo and replace things that were shifted, all the ongoing instructions, relentless repetition, getting involved in irrational arguments. Only after Dad went into care, which you'll hear about next, did some of her friends make comment on how much better she looked with some proper rest and a lot more sleep:

"There were a number of people at the dance that I know reasonably well, who a bit later on down the line, when they knew Bob had gone into care, had said, "Oh my God, you look so much better, you looked terrible, you looked so tired." So they all noticed. They didn't say anything until they knew that that's what happened. So, you know, all my thoughts about what people would think and all that sort of thing, really, they were just thinking, you know, probably it's a good thing because you look like you were going downhill."

In relation to the ongoing exhaustion, Mum reflects:

"It brought out a different side of me because I wasn't getting a lot of sleep...he wasn't sleeping through the night, and he was up and about... I became sleep deprived, certainly, but also angry, and I was finding it hard to, you know, to just watch what I was saying or not shout at him. And, you know, sometimes I would shout at him, and that would make him shout back at me. And that

was a different type of relationship to what it had been because, you know, Dad and I virtually didn't shout at one another in the normal relationship... And when that would happen, I would then feel terrible remorse, really awful about it afterwards and think that was a terrible thing to say or whatever."

Sadness – Despite the frustration, the anger, the sleep deprivation, and the ongoing challenges, as you would expect, there has always been a sadness about Dad's dementia:

"sadness for him because he'd always been such a ... you know, he was a farmer but he also flew a plane. He was very capable in his own self, and to think of him slowly getting to that stage, that was pretty sad."

"When I would calm down, or whatever the situation was, I think I could always get back to feeling sort of sad that I felt like I didn't know who he was anymore, and then thinking, well, you know, it's not his fault, he didn't ask to have dementia, that's the disease that's causing him to be like this. It's not that he's decided to be like this to annoy me... It's the unconditional love, and I think that I always managed to get back to that."

I'm aware there has been quite a negative focus on the information contained in this chapter, but I feel that has been necessary in painting a realistic picture of dementia and how hard things can get as the disease progresses. It's also important to say, things weren't always so difficult! Even after his formal diagnosis, things with Dad were quite manageable for Mum at home over a period of many, many months, really up until the point where his night-time disturbance became more and more intense, and he required an ever-increasing level of supervision. As you'll read in a later chapter, we remain very grateful for the years Dad lived at home with us, despite the challenges.

TAKE-HOME MESSAGE FROM THIS CHAPTER

Caring for someone with dementia at home can be very challenging, and there's a lot of trial and error in working out what the person can and can't do anymore, and then changing the approach as the disease progresses with time. And just like the carer role can be hard, so can managing the 'moving feast' of emotions that a dementia diagnosis throws up on an ongoing basis. Carers are not machines, and carer burnout is (almost) guaranteed, particularly if sleep deprivation is at play. Just like a new mother cannot give the best of herself to her baby if she's not addressing her self-care, it is the same for full-time carers of those with dementia — they cannot be to their loved one what they want to be if they're not getting replenishing sleep, regular time out, and/or respite. Although my husband and I supervised Dad at home, took him out with us again and again, and stayed with him overnight a few times so Mum could take a break, we were juggling home education, jobs, kids' activities, clients, friends, and so on, so we were never a true replacement for the 24/7 carer role Mum played.

None of us know how we'd cope in a full-time carer role until we (often unexpectedly) find ourselves in it. Similarly, looking in from the outside always offers a perspective not available to the people 'inside' the challenging situation, who are doing their best to manage their feelings and make sense of an ever-changing 'new normal'. I hope this chapter has raised your awareness, or perhaps validated your experience, of how significantly life can be changed with a dementia diagnosis. That's not to say it's all bad and there's no hope. If I believed that to be the case, I would never have had the drive to write this book 😊

CHAPTER TWO
COURAGE

"Fear is a reaction, courage is a decision"
– Winston Churchill

One of Dad's famous quotes is, "The easiest thing to do is to do nothing". This quote was often rolled out if you had approached him for advice when making a decision, particularly if that decision was going to take courage. It was his way of pointing out that although the easiest option is often the most attractive (because you don't need to change anything), it is not necessarily the best option. In other words, sometimes you just have to do really hard stuff. And so it was for us when the time came to change Dad's living arrangements and put him into full-time residential care. It was time to face our own fears, invite deep emotion into our lives, and do really hard stuff.

As you read in the previous chapter, it was becoming increasingly stressful for Mum having Dad at home, as he was steadily declining, his behaviours were becoming more challenging, and he required more supervision. What you haven't read yet, but what was made more complicated with the arrival of the pandemic, was that we had not really formulated a Plan B, though Mum and I had gone to view (only) one of the local facilities (where Dad now lives) three months earlier, "just to have a look". Mum certainly wasn't ready to consider care for Dad at that stage, though she did fill in an application form and agree to have his name put on their waiting list. At that time I had no intention of "pushing" Mum to change the status quo, mainly due to the relief we felt that Dad was at home as COVID ravaged nursing homes, people were locked in their rooms, and no one could visit. I also never wanted to be in the position of taking the decision away from Mum, however, I was becoming increasingly stressed and more and more worried about her well-being. I was constantly questioning myself about how much longer I would be comfortable leaving her in the primary carer role (in order to keep Dad at home), not only for her own sake but also due to the ongoing stress on Dad. I could see her deteriorating, and I could also see she was slowly but surely losing her natural kindness and empathy as she was consumed by the role of full-time carer.

Things came to a head one morning when I heard Mum highly distressed downstairs, shouting at Dad. I had the realisation the time had come for me to be brave, I had to step in and take control for everybody's sake. I joined her in the kitchen, burst into tears, and said, "Mum, you can't keep doing this". She was in tears as well. Then Dad was in tears because he could see both of us crying. He, of course, had no idea the distress was anything to do with him, and he was trying to comfort Mum in the best way he could. It was tough. I said, "Mum, it's time for us to do something different". It was probably one of the most difficult things I have ever had to do – effectively push my own mother to make a decision which would involve her no longer living with my dad, her husband of sixty plus years. As difficult as it was, my gut told me it was the right thing to do, and as I explain a little more in the upcoming chapter on guilt, I told Mum I was one hundred percent sure Dad would never resist moving into care if he had any insight into the fact that he was the reason she was so stressed out. I also suggested to Mum (and I think it helped) that if things were the other way around and I was watching Dad lose his mind looking after her on a full-time basis, she would definitely say to me, "Just tell him to put me somewhere else to be looked after".

What happened next could be described as either fate, intervention from the universe, or simply good timing, depending on how you view the world. We agreed I would make contact with the local facility, where we had put Dad's name down, to see where we were on the waitlist. We would reassess after we had their update. When I rang later that morning, the lady told me she was going to ring us that day as a bed had become vacant, and she wondered if we were interested in taking it for Dad. Woah, suddenly it was potentially a reality that he might be moving into care. Over the next couple of days, there were discussions and interstate phone calls between Mum, myself, and my brothers, and there were also plenty of tears. Mum knew that ultimately she had to make the decision herself, but she also knew there was now a viable Plan B, and she had the backing of her family to implement a new plan and go down a different pathway to what we had always imagined for Dad.

It was a difficult few days, and I'd like you to hear a little bit of Mum's reflection on how those days were for her:

> *"It was hard, and I wasn't very keen on the idea of putting him into care because we'd heard so much about aged care homes from people who already had others in there, and not real good stories about a lot of them… Also, the fact that I felt I would feel guilty if I had to put him into care… I think at the beginning when you first mentioned it, I wasn't ready for it – I don't know if I was ever ready for it really, but I certainly wasn't ready for it then. I was probably in denial that I couldn't cope and that I would be thinking about doing that. So I guess, in some ways, it was all to do with guilt on my part that I couldn't look after him myself. And fear that if I let him go in there, what was going to happen to him? Because, you know, I'd heard so many not-very-good stories about it… The other thing for me was that he'd had a couple of times of respite before that, and I could remember him saying the first time that he didn't really want to go. And, he said, "I don't want to be somewhere I don't know", and I knew he had a few of those fears in himself… And thinking that going into permanent care is different to going in for a fortnight's respite, I was frightened in my own self how that would pan out when we got there. How would I get him in there? But I suppose in amongst all that, after a little while, I could realise that you were right. I wasn't coping, and we couldn't go on the way we were, so something had to change."*

It took immense courage and it certainly wasn't easy for her, but, in the end, Mum reached the decision we should accept the vacancy being offered to Dad. The facility was very close to home, it presented well, it had a relatively "good vibe", they offered end-of-life care, and it was unknown when the next bed may become available if we didn't act now. She'd made what I knew in my heart was the right decision, albeit a decision I (in fact all of us) knew was about to deliver a massive test for that very same heart.

There were things to attend to over the next two weeks as we prepared to move Dad, and as you can imagine, it was a highly emotional time. One of Mum's greatest concerns was what to tell Dad, when to tell him, and what to do if he reacted in a negative way. As he was going to be admitted as a respite patient on a two-week trial initially, we ended up telling him he was going into respite again so that Mum could have a break (which he had last done in another facility several months earlier). Mum did harbour some guilt about lying to Dad (which was not something she was in the habit of doing), because we pretty much knew it was going to be permanent, barring a major catastrophe. But it seemed like the easiest way for all of us to handle it at the time, and we had to take the 'easy wins' where we could. Dad accepted the explanation and presented no challenge whatsoever on the day Mum moved him in. Thankfully he has been settled there from day one, even after he was moved into a high-care area a few weeks later. Although Mum worried for quite some time afterwards that he might reach a point of resistance to the new arrangement or even try and leave, Dad never asked about coming home, he never questioned the reason he'd gone into care, and he never complained. As teary as it still makes me to write this, even eighteen months later, he had already moved on from his days at home with his family and was immediately content in his new accommodation. Thank goodness for "living in the moment". It's been a massive comfort for the rest of us.

We always knew the day Dad entered care was going to be 'a high courage day', demanding a lot of inner strength. And to say it was difficult would be an understatement; it was terrible. But we were prepared for terrible and had put a plan in place for how to mitigate the terribleness. I had commitments out and about with the kids that morning, but I knew when Mum would be arriving back home after settling Dad in, and I obviously made sure I was there. As expected, there were floods of tears and our hearts were very heavy. It was particularly tough for Mum as she felt Dad's ongoing presence throughout the flat – it was quiet, there was no-one following her around, and his bed was empty. We had no choice but to back ourselves, draw on the strength we had used to get us that far, and stick to our inner belief (or call it gut instinct) that we were doing the right thing for both Mum and Dad. We had to sit with the discomfort of the changed arrangement until that discomfort eased and we were able to settle into the new normal, just like Dad had already done. There were certainly days in the lead-up to him going into care, and after the first few days he was there, when Mum wavered about her decision and wondered if she should take him out and bring him back home. And, of course, this was always to be expected and part of the grieving journey we were on at that moment in time.

Little did we know the next test of our courage and resolve was just around the corner. Less than a week after he went into care, we went into a state-wide COVID lockdown, meaning all our movements were restricted and no-one could visit Dad. This was both the best and worst thing that could have happened within the first few days. It was particularly devastating for Mum – she was racked with guilt, she was worried Dad would be upset and wondering why he was stuck in a place he didn't know, and also why she wasn't coming to visit. I was relatively confident he had passed the point of understanding timeframes, would be unaware when he had last seen anyone, and would not be thinking about where he used to live. But, nevertheless, it was upsetting to think of him stuck in a brand-new environment, with his already confused mind and with no access to a familiar face. The upside was that we did a heap of tidying up and sorting out, meaning it was quite a cathartic and somewhat restful time for Mum. As well as Dad being able to speak to Mum by phone when he was a little agitated, the other positive that came out of those first couple of weeks was that I was able to advocate for Mum to be part of the 'Partners in Care' initiative which had been introduced into his facility. This basically granted access to one family member who was prepared to go in (supposedly for an hour, though this wasn't really policed) and help deliver their loved one's care at a time when workforce shortages were placing huge demand on staffing levels. Although she had to wear full protective attire, at least it meant Mum could spend some time with Dad, she could see he was okay, and she felt like she was doing something to help him again. It also very much helped the rest of us who had no access to Dad at all during those restricted times, something that continued for many weeks. This arrangement has been such a blessing, as it has meant every time there has been a lockdown since, and there have been a number of them, Mum has always been allowed to visit and have face-to-face contact with Dad.

Thanks to the lockdown, which was imposed before I had even had a chance to visit (and the ongoing restrictions which followed), the first time I saw Dad again was many weeks after he had left home. I was desperate to see him by then, as you can probably imagine, and I knew it would be a significant test of my inner strength. We were still not allowed to take him out at that time, and the requirement for full personal protective equipment remained in place, so I gowned up, masked up, and in I went. I was elated to see him, and he was in a happy frame of mind, but it was a highly emotional afternoon for me, with a massive outpouring of tears afterwards. I managed to 'hold it together' while saying goodbye to him, but as soon as I left his area I was bawling. As well as the relief I felt at finally being able to visit, it was also a release of the realisation I had that Dad was never coming back to live at home. Of course there have been other days since when I've left him and had a similar response, particularly if he's been a bit down or seemed a bit more vulnerable than usual. At the end of the day, this stuff is hard. These are matters of the heart, and matters of the heart hurt (a lot) sometimes.

Before I sign off on this chapter, I'd like to share some final thoughts from Mum about the fears she faced and the courage she showed in deciding to put Dad into full-time care:

"To be truthful, I don't think the fear left. When I made that decision, I think the fear was still there. And the guilt was still there. I think the other thing that happened was the bed came up sooner than we expected it to... We didn't have long to make the definite decision – even though we'd made the decision earlier that we were going to put his name down, it came up much quicker than we thought... So that probably made it a bit harder, although maybe you could say that made it easier because if you had him here for longer, and we weren't sure when he was going to get a bed, and it was dragging on, that might have actually been harder. So, I don't know, certainly those feelings were still there even although I knew the decision was the right one...even if I was questioning afterwards whether I'd done the right thing with the lockdown and everything."

TAKE-HOME MESSAGE FROM THIS CHAPTER

As hard as it was to confront Mum that morning and tell her outright, "Something needs to change", I'm very glad I found the courage to do it. And at a time when she was exhausted and seeing a side of herself she didn't like (despite being fearful and full of guilt), I'm even more glad Mum had the courage to follow through and make a really difficult decision.

Sometimes you just need to be courageous, trust yourself, and do really hard stuff, no matter how much you may not want to or what the potential costs might be. For us it reached a stage where "doing nothing" was no longer a choice. We had to make a hard decision, and we also had to be prepared to feel a significant impact in our hearts as a result. Just like others have had to deal with the death of a child, a move away from family or friends, a decision to turn off a life support machine, clawing their way back from financial ruin, or leaving a marriage, we had to dig deep and be brave, assuming there would be a benefit a little further down the line.

Sometimes you need to embrace the hard moments and trust in yourself to get out the other side of it. I have always taken great comfort in the fact that Dad has been settled in care from day one and has never refused to go back after being out with us. And in the meantime, I've got my Mum back. She is back to being able to enjoy her time with Dad and make the most of her time with him, as opposed to feeling overwhelmed and stressed by her full-time caring role. She is also free to do other things she enjoys with us and her friends whenever she likes – that is the silver lining that courage has delivered.

> **"Listen to your inner voice. Trust your intuition. It's important to have the courage to trust yourself"**
> **– Dawn Ostroff**

CHAPTER THREE
GUILT

"Guilt is the thief of life" – Anthony Hopkins

Guilt is a very personal thing, and it's something that has manifested itself quite differently for Mum and I as we have gone through this experience with Dad. Some thoughts from Mum first:

There's the guilt that follows diagnosis:

There were the thoughts of:

> *"Why us? Isn't my cancer and the financial stressors we've had in our life enough? What about all the things we're not going to be able to do or have anymore and all the plans we had…? How will it affect our relationship…?"*

And then her follow-up guilt about even having such thoughts:

> *"…because plenty of people have more to worry about than that."*

There's the ongoing guilt about the (unplanned) full-time carer role:

Feeling frustrated at not being able to go for coffee or to a movie with a friend, and then feeling guilty because:

> *"that's not a very nice way of thinking when Bob has dementia."*

There's plenty of guilt around the feeling of not coping:

"Guilt that I'm not doing my role very well.

Guilt that I'm thinking I can't do this and therefore I might have to send him off to somewhere else for someone else to look after.

Guilt that I'm not understanding where he is, because I don't know a lot about dementia. Some of these behaviours, you know, that I'm yelling at him about or that I'm not understanding.

Guilt about the fact that maybe I should be able to work this out better and be more of a help to him than I think I am at the moment.

Guilt and terrible remorse after I said something horrible to him."

And then came the guilt associated with putting Dad into care:

"I'm Bob's wife, I should be able to look after him no matter what is wrong with him because that's part of my role.

What are my friends going to think about me not coping and putting Bob into care?

What will he think? I didn't think he'd like the idea, and I thought he would think I was trying to get rid of him."

Is the guilt still there?

"I think there's still a bit there sometimes, depending on how he is. It's getting less because I can see now that Bob's certainly in the moment, and he's quite happy to be where he is."

These feelings of guilt can be quickly reignited, however, when Mum fronts up to visit and things are not how she expected them to be:

"Like when he's lying there and he's still got his pyjamas on, he hasn't had a shave, and, you know, he just looks neglected. And I think, it wouldn't be like this if he was at home... Still that sort of little thought, which is stupid I know, because I know he's being well looked after. Or if he doesn't seem all that happy, I wonder if something's happened... But then I come away and think to myself, there's no point in feeling guilty about that because whatever it was or whatever it is, the next time I go, you'll be fully dressed, you'll be ready to come out, and you'll be quite happy. So, one day at a time, you never know what's going to be there when you go there. But yeah, there are certainly still some times when I feel a little bit guilty."

Mum and I have talked about these lingering feelings of guilt and how easily they bubble up to the surface again and again. To some extent, I think they could also just be natural feelings of protectiveness toward someone who is increasingly vulnerable – a similar kind of feeling we have toward our children when we're watching them battle illness or suffering in some way. The most important thing for Mum is that the guilt is slipping away as time passes.

At the point Dad passes away, can you imagine you will be able to let go of any remaining guilt?

"I think so, yeah, if it's even still there when he passes away... it's a lot less. I think I'll be really sad when he's gone and he's not here anymore, but I won't feel guilt that we didn't have him here because I think we've put him in the right place where he needed to be, and we've done as much as we can while he's been in there to try and keep him happy. So, I think that's how it'll be, and I'll feel quite peaceful."

Quite peaceful. We can't ask for anything more than that.

And now onto my own thoughts about guilt… Did I feel guilty about putting Dad into care?

No. As difficult as that day was, and it was very difficult, the one thing I did not really experience around that time was guilt. I had an overwhelming belief that if I had been able to have ten minutes of complete clarity with Dad (which by then I couldn't) and say to him, "Dad, Mum's really struggling having you at home 24/7, 'cause it's really hard looking after you when you need so much help", I just KNEW he'd say, "put me into care Lee, but (with a sparkle in his eye and a smirk on his face) don't bloody forget about me, make sure you come and see me". This feeling gave me great strength in the lead-up to him entering care, as well as on the day he moved in, and it also enabled me to cope with the immense sadness I felt knowing Dad would never live at home with us all again.

So what did I feel guilty about?

Interestingly enough, the guilt I felt as we have gone through this journey has actually been in relation to Mum, not Dad. As Dad's disease progressed and he became more and more vulnerable, I felt increasingly protective of him and, subsequently, increasingly frustrated and angry with Mum when she was short-tempered and impatient toward him. Having to confront my own mother about her lack of tolerance with Dad was both stressful and upsetting. I felt guilty about it every time. I KNEW how hard her role was, but I couldn't help myself as it was causing me great distress too. I would debrief to one of my brothers or my husband, and then I would feel awful for talking about Mum in such a negative manner. I wasn't the one who was up with him all night, it wasn't me helping him in the shower, repeating myself all day long, being shadowed by him everywhere I went, or having to stop him from doing something. Yes I was around and helping out some of the time, but I was not in the primary caring role she was in, and I was not "on-call" twenty-four hours a day. On all those occasions I confronted Mum and told her she needed to be more patient, more understanding, and more empathetic, she could certainly have been forgiven for thinking I was not only criticising her but also indirectly suggesting I could do better myself. And I'm very sure that wasn't pleasant for her. I'm a parent, I've had those experiences where someone (often a random stranger) suggests you should have handled a situation with your children differently or leaves you in no doubt they are judging you in a negative way. I know the feelings of guilt and failure this can evoke, and I felt guilty I was doing the same to my Mum, who was just trying her best in a very difficult situation. I'm pleased to say I don't harbour that guilt anymore, but it was real and it was uncomfortable at the time. I'm even more pleased to say my relationship with Mum has not suffered as a result of our experience with Dad, and if anything, it has probably brought us closer as we've ridden this rollercoaster together.

Final thoughts about guilt?

We'll never know whether our situation would have panned out any differently if the COVID pandemic hadn't come along – would we have considered putting Dad into care earlier if we hadn't had images on our screens night after night of the elderly dying in record numbers in nursing homes? Would caring for Dad at home have been any easier on Mum without restrictions, lockdowns, and ongoing worry about getting sick affecting their options for getting out and about? Would we have pushed for the increase in Dad's in-home support package to be expedited (for which he'd already been approved prior to entering care) if Mum had felt more open to workers coming in and out of the house? We can speculate on all these things and many more, but it doesn't change anything, and it achieves nothing. One thing I can say though, is that the pandemic was only **one** of the things that increased the pressure Mum felt to keep Dad at home and struggle through.

The other major thing was the fact that we'd never really formulated a Plan B. Right from the beginning we'd talked about Dad staying at home, we'd made a few minor modifications in their granny flat, and we felt relief Dad wouldn't need to see out his days in a nursing home. Dad had always said he didn't want to go into care, because he found nursing homes miserable to visit, so we imagined a gradual increase in support and respite, leading up to the point where end-of-life care would be delivered at home. And this is very consistent with the messaging around aged care, in Australia at least, where people are encouraged to stay in their homes for as long as possible. Don't get me wrong, as a general rule I believe that idea has merit, and we're fortunate in-home support is an option in this country (though the system for delivering it has some well-documented issues). What I am saying though, is that this pressure definitely added to the expectation and feelings of responsibility Mum felt to cope with the situation she was in. It also added to the guilt she felt when she wasn't coping, some of which was (misplaced) guilt about what my brothers and I might have thought if she suggested putting Dad into care, given we had always imagined avoiding this scenario.

This is REALLY HARD stuff for primary carers to process, and all we can do is try not to be too harsh on ourselves and others. We are all learning as we go along (and as the disease changes our loved ones), and we must constantly remind ourselves we are doing the best we can in the circumstances we are in right then.

TAKE-HOME MESSAGE FROM THIS CHAPTER

Guilt has been part of our journey with Dad, and I suspect it's part of most people's journey with sickness and disease, in some format. It feels heavy, and it can be hard to get rid of. The thing about guilt, and the reason it does not serve you to harbour it for a long time, is that everyone is different – yet we tend to compare ourselves to others, assume what they think of us, judge ourselves accordingly, and then experience (often misplaced) guilt. But we all have different thresholds for managing situations, we come at life from different perspectives, and we can't ever truly know how we would act in a given situation. We should, therefore, not compare. "Comparison is the thief of joy", as Theodore Roosevelt is quoted as saying.

Whilst we've all had times where we've acted in a way we regretted later or felt guilty about upon reflection, it doesn't necessarily make us a bad person. I read a great quote about guilt once, which was something along the lines of "Although your behaviour may have been less than ideal, it doesn't define who you are". That is actually much more accurately defined by your own self-worth, your intentions, and how you support others.

CHAPTER FOUR
LIVING IN THE MOMENT

"Living in the moment is good enough"
– as spoken by my friend Susan B

As his illness progressed, Dad reached the inevitable point where he could ONLY live in the moment. It wasn't an active choice he was making; the choice was taken away from him as his cognitive function declined. I remember the first time I fully understood the notion of "living in the moment" as it pertains to someone with dementia. I realised my dad could no longer recall very much from the past and he also had no concept of the future. In other words, he could only "be" in the present, which was literally this second – he'd already forgotten what happened five minutes ago, and he had no understanding of what was about to happen (even if we had just discussed that with him a minute earlier, and probably five minutes before that). This also meant he reached a point where it wouldn't occur to him to anticipate something that needed to be done, nor would he be likely to offer his help in some way (because he couldn't notice any need for it). It wasn't that he didn't care anymore; he simply no longer had the capacity to behave as he would have in the past, due to the impact of the disease on his brain.

This concept of "living in the moment" has been one of the hardest things for Mum to understand, particularly after Dad went into care, and it took her quite a long time to get past it. She would come home from visiting him and say things like, "he's not asking to come back home", "he's not asking how you guys are", and "he doesn't ask me to stay". It actually felt quite hurtful to her, after being his primary carer for a few years prior to that, and she found it difficult to take on the idea that he didn't remember the house he used to live in, he wasn't hankering to get back there, and we were not front-of-mind for him anymore.

But, although I've come to an understanding of the concept at a "head level", there's certainly been occasions where Dad's "living in the moment" has had a full-on collision with my heart. Not that long ago for instance, more than eighteen months after he went into care, Mum had been visiting Dad at his care facility and was preparing to leave as his dinner was arriving. She said to him, "Okay, well I'll go now Bob", and he turned around and said to her, "But I don't want you to go". Mum managed to say that she was going home to have her dinner too, then rushed outside and burst into tears. When she arrived home, she said to me, "Oh my god, when I went to go, Dad said he didn't want me to leave". Bang! Out of the blue the inner empathy button got pressed, and we were both in tears. At the end of the day, it's hard not to be moved by someone's expression of raw vulnerability.

Anyway, after we both settled, I was able to say to her, "Mum, Dad lives in the moment, and obviously right in that moment he thought, 'It's nice to have you here while I'm eating my dinner'. But, five minutes later, he would have forgotten you were even there, so it's okay. It's okay". And I took comfort in the fact I KNEW it would be okay, because the moment had passed, and he would have moved on. There have been other occasions when Dad has dissolved into tears, and it hasn't necessarily been obvious what prompted those tears to fall. Perhaps they stemmed from inner frustration or a brief insight into his situation, perhaps they were tears of loss, perhaps he was moved by another resident's obvious suffering, or perhaps he was simply in pain. Regardless of how that has tugged at our heart strings, the best we have been able to offer him in those moments is our presence, our love, and our connection. Just being comfortable to have a few tears ourselves and sit with him "in the moment".

In preparing to write this book, I interviewed a friend of mine, Susan, whose parents have both lived with dementia, and she reiterated the point that we, as family members, need to accept "living in the moment is good enough". She was explaining how her dad loves to potter in the garden, often just repetitively staying in one corner, and that you can talk to him, and he'll respond with something about his plants. She said, "I always go up to him and ask, 'Are you okay?' And he goes, 'I'm in my own world'. And when he says that, I know he's happy, you don't have to worry about him". She went on to recount a conversation she had with his doctor, who said, "They're in their own world, you don't have to worry about them because if they've got something to say, they will say it. But they're happy doing what they're doing, repetitive or not. Whether or not you sit there and go, 'Oh my God, look what they're doing', they're happy doing what they're doing. Leave them alone; that gives them peace". Who could begrudge someone a sense of peace if that's where they are positioned, particularly if they are living in the confusing world of dementia?

TAKE-HOME MESSAGE FROM THIS CHAPTER

Dementia is a terminal illness, and just like any other terminal illness, there is a sense of being "on a downhill slide", which follows diagnosis. No-one can tell you how long the slide is, how quickly you'll progress from one "stage" to the next, or whereabouts on the slide you are by the time an official diagnosis happens. **Just like those with dementia are "living in the moment", we should all try to live a bit more for today. Or, at the very least, we should try not to dwell on the past or worry so much about the future. We should put more effort into actively listening when people are talking to us, play when our kids ask us to, and put our phones away when we are surrounded by natural beauty. Truly living in the moment has the capacity to deliver inner peace and a little more calmness to all of us, not just our loved ones who are challenged by dementia.**

CHAPTER FIVE
GRATITUDE

"If you cannot find gratitude, you'll never find peace"
– Leticia Rae

Gratitude may not be a "life lesson" that springs to mind in this context, but actually, there are a number of things I'm super grateful for in terms of Dad's journey with dementia.

Dad is teaching our kids empathy, kindness, tolerance, inclusiveness, acceptance

Our children are growing up with dementia very much part of their lives. They are home-educated, so they've been around and about Mum and Dad constantly since the ages of three and four. They are witnessing Dad's decline, just like the rest of us, as he slowly but surely succumbs more and more to the disease. When Dad still lived at home, I would often take him with me to collect the kids from an external class or to transport them here and there. Sometimes he'd walk into their art class, pick whatever he saw up, and make a comment about it. Or he might laugh inappropriately at something on the drive, or miss a social cue when we were talking to someone whilst out and about. But the kids wouldn't express embarrassment or humiliation, and they never asked me not to bring him. They knew Dad had dementia, many others around them knew he had dementia, and there was nothing more to say, no judgement to be made.

They were learning to take things in their stride and just roll with the crazy punches dementia can deliver. Unlike Dad's other grandchildren, who were born a lot earlier than our kids, their main memories of him, and connection to him, have been since he has been challenged by memory loss and cognitive decline. They have had to learn to slow down and be patient with Dad; they've had to learn it's okay if you don't understand what he's saying around the lunch table (because it doesn't make sense anymore) or what he's laughing about to himself; and it's okay that he repeats his questions over and over again. They've had to accept he doesn't always acknowledge them if he's in his own world when they appear. They've had to steer him to the table, which he knows so well, when he's headed off in the wrong direction. And they've also had to witness how hard it was on Mum, in particular, to care for him when she was in a sleep-deprived, highly stressed state. They've seen the tears from Mum and me many times. They know the reality of his decline, and they understand why we prioritise simple outings with him over other invitations at times.

I simply cannot view any of that from a position other than gratitude, and I strongly believe there is no greater gift we could have given our children than instilling in them a sense of empathy, kindness, tolerance, and acceptance. In the words of Ben Franklin, "Tell me and I forget. Teach me and I remember. Involve me and I learn". They are learning from their involvement with Dad.

For much of the COVID-19 pandemic, Dad lived at home

As you have already read, Mum and Dad were living at home with us for just over five years prior to diagnosis, and Dad remained there for another three and a half years afterwards. This meant we had him with us for a large part of the pandemic, certainly throughout the time that was so deadly for elderly nursing home residents. Although by then things were getting increasingly stressful for Mum, and the role of 24/7 carer was taking a heavy toll on her, truth be told, Dad could well have passed away, alone, if he had been in care during the worst months of COVID. He is prone to chest infections and pneumonia, so this would not have been outside the realm of possibilities – look how many aged care residents did pass away, including many who were in good health previously. To this day, my heart still breaks for everyone who had family members with dementia in care or living at home alone during that prolonged period of time.

Mum and Dad were at least able to get out in the yard, use the backyard pool, go for a walk locally, eat outside, and have our ongoing support. Not only did we have peace of mind that they were safe in their own environment and could still enjoy some family connection, but my (interstate) brothers could rest easy in the knowledge they were with me, my husband, and our kids. I cannot tell you how grateful we all are for our situation during those times, and that sense of gratitude will never leave me. As you already heard, when a bed did become available at a facility close by, and although we have had to deal with lockdowns and restrictions a number of times since, Dad was basically settled from day one. And we have never had the experience of him trying to leave or refusing to go back after he has been with us at home for the day. In fact, it's usually Dad who will say something like "I think it's time to be going back now" when he feels ready to return to his care facility. That has been a great comfort for our family, and we consider ourselves very lucky on that front.

We could have lost him (more than once), and the (new) lesson we learnt each time

One day Dad set off to attend a funeral eleven kilometres away. This was prior to diagnosis; he was still driving, and he should have been familiar with the route. He never made it to the funeral; instead, he headed in the wrong direction and was gone for many hours. He had no idea where he was and could not explain his location (which kept changing) to Mum over the phone. We had no way of tracking him – a Smartphone was something he was unable to manage by that stage (so he just had his 'old clunker'), and he wasn't wearing a GPS-equipped watch. When he finally made it safely home late in the day, he couldn't really explain to us where he had been, but with what we could piece together, it was obvious he had covered many, many kilometres and was a long way off course. It seems he had asked a few people along the way for directions but had been unable to follow them. One thing we came to understand, however, was that some very kind soul had worked out the problem and took the time to escort Dad (driving in front of him in their own car) onto the motorway, headed in a direction he then, thankfully, clearly recognised would lead him home. Lesson learned – that was the last time Dad was allowed to drive anywhere other than the very local destinations he knew extremely well – the supermarket, the newsagent, the Men's Shed, the GP.

We had another alarming incident with Dad after he had surrendered his license at diagnosis, this time on foot. Mum had gone out, and the kids and I were coming and going from the house on and off throughout the day, as had happened many times at that stage. Dad had never been a 'wanderer', and the only place he would usually walk would be up to the shop to buy the paper (little more than five hundred metres away). Perhaps he remembered that Mum had left by train that day, who knows, but he wandered down to the station (very close to our house) and took a train ride. We never quite got to the bottom of where he went, but once again, when we were piecing his movements together afterwards, it seemed like one of the railway staff took the time to assess his situation, check his 'swipe on' location, and determine that he should probably return to the station he came from, at which point he arrived back home just after we had started looking for him around the local area. Lesson learned – that was the last time Dad was ever left home alone. When we went out, he either went with one of us, or we 'tag teamed' throughout the day, depending on who was going where. Thankfully Dad was always happy to tag along, no matter how boring the task, how long the drive, or the time of day!

The two final (scary) incidents happened on the last holiday Mum and Dad took together on their own. Having given up their big travel plans several years earlier when it was obvious these would no longer suit Dad's declining capacities, they decided to take a two-week road trip (Mum driving by then) in regional Queensland. It seemed very manageable with how Dad was at the time, and we thought we had mitigated all potential issues with good planning. Things went along swimmingly until close to the end of the trip, and then it happened. Mum locked up the hotel when they went to bed and woke up to police knocking on the door with Dad. He got up during the night, unbeknown to her, felt unfamiliar with his surroundings, and wandered outside. Sigh of relief – someone had seen him, called the police, and he was returned. Mum was extremely shaken, as you can imagine, and we agreed they should abandon the rest of the trip and just make their way back home. As they were too far away for Mum to drive the return journey in one day, they had to make it through one more overnight stay. This time, Mum barricaded the front door with furniture when she locked up; however, Houdini (aka Dad) moved it to the side and once again wandered off during the night when his surroundings were unfamiliar. This time when Mum realised he was gone and raised the alarm with hotel staff, the Special Emergency Services were called in to search for him. Ironically, he was in another room of the hotel, sleeping soundly away despite the panic. Lesson learned – the holiday was over. My husband and I packed the kids into the car, drove four hundred kilometres to meet them, and brought them home safely. As you can see, we have a LOT to be grateful for in each of those scenarios, because every single one of them could have ended tragically.

You have to be able to have a laugh!

Dad has always had a good sense of humour, and I can safely say, so have the rest of us! Just as well, because something we have all learnt as we've travelled down the path of dementia is that it's VITAL to maintain a sense of humour and be able to roll with the craziness at times. That's everything from Dad pretending to do wheelies with his walking frame; to the funny faces and expressions he has made (which may or may not have been appropriate for the moment); to the time Mum was ordering take-away pizza and looked around to find Dad was starting to take his clothes off behind her; to the funny coloured, sparkling hats he has taken to wearing everywhere (including in bed) and odd clothing combinations he has donned at times; to the fake tears and proclamation of "boo hoo" he made as my brother was saying goodbye before heading back to South Australia last year.

He has mimicked us when we have inadvertently said something apparently patronising to him. He has smashed unshelled nuts apart with a hammer because he didn't believe he could eat them as they were. He even went into a friend's bathroom, got in their shower in the middle of the night, and put the other man's clothes on (when Mum and Dad were sharing a weekend away with them), completely unperturbed in the morning. In his care facility, there's been an ongoing parade of other residents' shoes, socks, clothes, and mementoes- just as many of his things have been seen in the possession of others, regardless of whether or not they are a good fit or suitable for the occasion. It's all the funny little things, and there've been many, many of them, that can lighten the mood, offer a circuit breaker when things are stressful, and provide a glimpse into Dad's personality, which I'm so grateful to have shared with him as we are moving through the stages of his dementia.

Thank goodness we took that family trip

Back in mid-2019 (about eighteen months post-diagnosis), my eldest brother suggested we try and coordinate a family trip back to Dad's childhood home area in New South Wales, while he was still capable of making the journey. This was not the simplest of suggestions (with that brother in South Australia, my other brother in Western Australia, us in Queensland, all 3 of us working, our kids being home-educated, and Dad's decreasing capacity for change, his insomnia, etc.); however, we pulled it all together in October that year, and it was ABSOLUTELY FANTASTIC. Not only was this the first time in many years we had spent time together just as a family of five, but it was also the first time we had all been together since Dad's diagnosis. There were opportunities for tears, frank discussions, reassurance, support, plenty of laughs, and even more food!! I will be forever grateful to my brother for suggesting we make that trip (a few months later and we would have been completely blocked by ongoing border closures), and also to my husband and friends who took care of the kids to make it happen from our end.

Upon our return, I put together a photo book of the trip for each of us, and it's something that brings all of us, including Dad, for whom family has always been very important, great comfort and happiness whenever we look through it. Having spoken to a friend whose sister stole money from her mother after she (her mother) was diagnosed with dementia, I am eternally grateful we have never been in a situation of family or sibling conflict as we have managed Dad's dementia. Despite being spread across the country, we have all been working towards the same goal – a good end to a happy life for Dad.

Knowledge is power

Like many people who face health challenges, I went to Google for help, assurance, and hope in the early days. I read about alternative treatments for dementia (a couple of which we tried), and I had a need to educate myself (and Mum) about the potential road ahead, what resources there were (helplines, newsletters, publications), and so on. No-one in the family had much knowledge about dementia prior to Dad displaying symptoms, so we were in quite unfamiliar territory, so to speak. It's fair to say the lack of information meant it was hard for Mum, in particular, not to feel frustrated or angry with Dad about his responses, his behaviour, him losing things, his repetitive questions, and so on. Sometime during the first year post-diagnosis, my friend Kathy told me she had completed a free online course about dementia (details about the course are contained in a later chapter), and she recommended it to me. I am so grateful she did, and I have since recommended it to several other people for whom I thought it would be useful. Although I had done some reading about dementia prior to undertaking the course, this was the kind of resource I needed. It suited my learning style and what I had capacity for at the time – lots of videos, simple slides, real-life snippets, audio, etc. As I worked my way through the material, I was able to share much of it with Mum, and my husband went on and completed the course as well. Knowledge is power, and I applaud the University of Tasmania for making this course free and accessible to anyone who wants to enrol in it, anywhere in the world.

**"Fear comes from the lack of knowledge and a state of
ignorance. The best remedy for fear is to gain knowledge"
– Debasish Mridha**

The simple things in life are (very often) the best

Simplicity means a lot to someone who has ever-decreasing options, both physically and mentally. This journey with Dad has been a good reminder to prioritise what (and who) is important, to think about how you measure success and happiness, and to get back to basics – he doesn't need complicated, he doesn't need fancy, he doesn't need expensive. To be honest, he's never needed those things and has often quoted a man he knew whose motto was "Never make money your God". Dad loves his family and just wants to be included, to sit around the table with everyone else, unwrap a Christmas present, have something nice to eat, throw something into the conversation (whether or not it makes sense), and be loved and respected for the person who's still inside. Especially as he has declined more and more, it's forced us to make sure that, whilst ever he still can, he has the opportunity to experience the simple pleasure that comes from things like sitting by the beach, watching small children playing by the water, feeling the sun, receiving a validating smile from others who walk past, an afternoon tea picnic, or watching dogs in their happy place at the beach. These are the kinds of things that still bring him joy, and we don't know how many of those moments we have left. Not knowing her mother was going to unexpectedly pass away, my friend Susan told me how blessed she felt that she set up an iPad for her mother, so they could see each other and cook dinner together, despite being thousands of kilometres apart, also commenting that "every conversation with her is going to be treasured". These experiences have provided great comfort to Susan since her mother's death – the simple things in life are often the best.

**"May you always value the simple little things in life.
For they make a big difference and hence are the most
important." – Omar Cherif**

TAKE-HOME MESSAGE FROM THIS CHAPTER

Gratitude is something we can probably all get better at recognising and expressing. I'm writing this book at the end of the COVID pandemic, and I think the global experience did raise the "profile" of gratitude for a while there. **But the key to remaining in a grateful state is in recognising things to feel grateful for each and every day.** Some days that's harder than others; some days it feels almost impossible when times are tough and life feels relentless, but I can honestly say **Dad going through dementia has taught me there is always SOMETHING (and often many things) to be grateful for, if you're prepared to look.**

I started keeping a gratitude journal quite some time ago, and what I have written in there has often been very simple:

- sitting by the water with Dad, people or dog watching

- getting my washing dry on a winter's day

- receiving a thoughtful text from a friend saying just what I needed to hear in that moment

- the kids doing something helpful around the house without being asked

- reading in bed next to my husband at night

- noticing a beautiful sunset as I went to close the curtains

- getting a bargain at the supermarket…

There are opportunities for gratefulness all around us. Sometimes we just have to open our eyes (and our hearts) to find them.

CHAPTER SIX

NO REGRETS

"In the end…we only regret the chances we didn't take,
and the decisions we waited too long to make"
– Lewis Carroll

At the time of writing, Dad is almost 87, and none of us know how much longer he will live. But one thing I already know, and for which I am very grateful, is that I will have no regrets when he passes away. You may wonder how I can confidently say this, given death throws up all kinds of emotions people are not prepared for, and it's a fair question. I believe the reason I know is because of two things – **connection and intention**. I'll break that down for you.

The power of childhood connection

Put simply, if you're well connected to someone from your childhood, it's actually pretty easy to give a stuff about them and want the best for them! I've always felt a strong connection to my Dad. Growing up on a farm in the '70s, I can tell you he wasn't what would be referred to now as "a new-age dad". He didn't change our nappies, do the household washing, buy the groceries, or tell me he loved me every day. But I have never judged him by those parameters, and they are not important to me when I think of his role in my life. He was a wheat and sheep farmer, he worked the land and provided for his family. That's how it was in the '60s, '70s, and '80s when my brothers and I were growing up. However, what he has always been is open-minded, available for advice, supportive of our ideas, proud of our achievements, interested in our lives, and encouraging of our pursuits. Those are the qualities he has brought to parenting, and those are the reasons I have never once doubted how much he loved all three of us.

Dad's always been a significant person in my life, he was my go-to person for many years, and his opinion and advice are things I've always valued. So when something like dementia comes along, and the connection is strong, maybe it makes it easier to do things for your loved one? Because you WANT to do it; you're not doing it out of obligation. You still care greatly for that person, and it's very important to you what happens to them. You try to make the right decisions on their behalf. You go along with whatever needs to happen at a given time. And you feel okay about compromising on some things for yourself if this will be better for them. Don't get me wrong, there have been times when it has been quite confronting to watch his decline, especially recently, and he hasn't been able to act in a traditional fatherly role for a number of years now. However, he is still my Dad, and that won't change regardless of what happens from here.

Intention – we have purposely chosen to pursue 'a good end to life' for Dad

We have tried to focus on the things we can control, knowing we cannot control the disease affecting his brain. As you read in the chapter about the carer's emotional journey, this has been unbelievably hard at times, especially for Mum. But even when caring for him at home was at its toughest, there was never any doubt we were all working toward the same goal of trying to make the final years of Dad's life as meaningful and peaceful as possible. In our case, that meant making the excruciatingly difficult decision to put Dad into residential care a few years post-diagnosis. But we made that very intentional decision based on a need to preserve Mum's well-being and return her to a place where she could enjoy her time with Dad again.

TAKE-HOME MESSAGE FROM THIS CHAPTER

Our experience with dementia has really brought home to me how powerful childhood family connections can dramatically affect what happens much later in life. Like many other situations, it has also clearly highlighted to me that nothing is absolute – goalposts do move, decisions do need constant review, and options do change. **As long as your intention is to do what seems like the right thing in the circumstances, you should feel confident in the choices you make and the actions you take. And you should be able to avoid experiencing regret for what could or should have been.** I'll be very sad when Dad passes away and he's not around anymore, but I won't be sad due to regret about something we didn't do for him. That's one thing I am very sure of, and that feels calm and peaceful.

CHAPTER SEVEN

A FEW FINAL LESSONS

Kindness

> **"Wherever there is a human being,**
> **there is an opportunity for kindness"**
> **– Lucius Annaeus Seneca**

I'm sure you remember how, in the early stages of the COVID pandemic, a global kindness movement emerged, as people from all walks of life were forced into situations they had never dealt with before, had no knowledge of, and were fearful about. "Kindness matters" became a catchphrase for many, and it was screen-printed on clothing, projected onto buildings, and written on handmade signs honouring essential workers. The pandemic has now been declared officially over, but the need for human kindness remains!

And kindness matters a lot to someone who is no longer able to live their life the way they used to. Someone who can no longer understand things or behave in a way they used to, because they are challenged with dementia. They didn't ask for dementia, they can't help the fact they have dementia, and they have no control over their dementia. Their behaviours may be new, very different, and worrying, but you have to be able to step back and view them from the point of view of someone who is no longer able to process their thoughts and reactions in the same way they used to. One of the easiest things to offer someone with dementia is good old-fashioned kindness – it costs nothing, it cuts through their layers of mental confusion, and it has the magical effect of making you feel good about yourself in return. Don't hold back, hand it out by the bucket load.

Time

"Time is the most valuable thing a man can spend"
- Theophrastus

My yoga teacher always opens her class by encouraging us to "put aside the busyness, the doing, and the rushing". That's to encourage us to 'stay present' and focus on our breath and inner self as we go through the practice, but it's also relevant advice when it comes to giving our time to others. Just like most other families I know, our lives get busy too – with home education, teenagers in the house, extra-curricular activities, shift work, clients, volunteer roles, and so on, it's almost impossible not to have some busy days, or even some busy weeks. But we do prioritise time with Dad over other things whenever we can, and we always make the most of our time whenever we are with him. Thankfully, at this stage, he is still able to watch our dog playing at the beach or come home for lunch or afternoon tea, and we particularly value those moments we have, sitting around the table together like we so often have. These experiences always remind me that none of us know how much time we have left, or how much time the others around us have. It's so important to prioritise it, make the most of it, and use it wisely, because we'll never get it back.

Acceptance (of others')

"Happiness can exist only in acceptance"
– George Orwell

One of the hardest lessons I have had to learn as we have gone through this journey with Dad is that not everyone in his previous life has had the capacity to 'stay the course' and deal with his dementia. Even people he has known for many decades have effectively removed themselves from his life, assumedly due to their own fears or lack of coping abilities. I have tried to model compassionate, inclusive behaviour rather than attempt to change the behaviour of others, so I have found this issue to be extremely confronting on many occasions, and I've harboured a great deal of anger about it at times. Probably because she's felt a degree of hurt herself, Mum has actually been the most useful in steering me through these situations, helping me reach the point where I could move on from my anger and see people's withdrawal from Dad as their loss, not his. Their way of handling things being very different to mine. Their understanding of the circumstances being very unlike ours. As Mum reminded me:

"Everyone deals with it in their own way. You're dealing with it in your way, and you shouldn't judge others. You need to meet them where they're at. Just like you've learnt your lessons, they'll learn theirs and reflect in their own way".

As painful as this facet of the journey has been for me at times, it has reminded me that it's important to accept other people's limitations. Not everyone has the same personal or professional skills to embrace change, adapt to change and learn from change. Perhaps it'll be easier for my generation (than my parents' generation) to accept when their friends are challenged by dementia? Sheer numbers of people being diagnosed suggests there should be less shame and stigma in coming generations, as the general community becomes more aware of the disease and, therefore, less fearful of it. Learning from my dad's experience about the way some have chosen to deal with him has been a tough lesson, but I finally reached a place of acceptance, understanding, and peace, for which I'm very grateful. Holding onto anger is never a healthy option, and I'm thankful I am no longer in that space. As Mum wisely made me see, if others had been able to stay in touch with him:

"...they would have been able to see that even though he's not the same Bob that he was, that they knew, he's still involved with us and would have enjoyed their company. So they've had that loss... we've been able to still be with him and, you know, see him like he is and still love him and all the rest of it. They haven't had that".

Don't sweat the small stuff

**"Ask yourself this question: Will this
matter a year from now?"
– Richard Carlson**

As I'm sure you've worked out while you made your way through this book, life can get challenging for those caring for someone with dementia, whether that's at home or in a care facility. One of the things dementia can throw up, and it did in our case, is a decreased ability to understand 'norms' – in our case it was often around dressing, namely clothes and shoes. Apart from when he was working on the farm (and often covered in dirt, grain husks, diesel, etc.), Dad had always presented in a neat and tidy fashion and would only EVER wear his pyjamas when he was literally climbing into bed. So, it will probably come as no surprise to hear how it has often felt rather strange whenever we have seen Dad with pyjamas over his clothes, shorts over his long pants, jackets on in bed, or odd shoes and socks at different times throughout the day. On those occasions where he has done his best to get himself dressed (perhaps thinking it will save someone else the trouble), it's always been important to question, 'Does it really matter right at this moment?'

Obviously we have wanted to maintain his dignity as much as possible, so if he was going out and about or someone was visiting, we may have gently persuaded him to make a change (similarly if he was dressed inappropriately for the weather). Otherwise, we have tried to remember not to 'sweat the small stuff' at times like this, to reduce the stress around simple things like him choosing his own clothes. Similarly, when he has been unable to accept an explanation about something (a good example was when his license was removed, and he insisted it was unfairly taken away due to his age), it has usually been easier not to continue arguing back and simply allow him to maintain his belief and move on when he's ready.

Advocacy

"All advocacy is, at its core, an exercise in empathy"
– Samantha Power

Fortunately for me (even if it's not ALWAYS been a positive!), I inherited some of my dad's bolshiness, stubbornness, and "dog with a bone" type attitude. He always stood up for himself and questioned unfair treatment or decisions he didn't agree with, so I guess it's in my blood! A desire to help people and advocate for the vulnerable is probably what drew me to the profession of Social Work in the first place, and, in this context, advocating for Dad has been very important to me, particularly as he's become more vulnerable and can't stand up for himself anymore. Whether that's been in relation to his in-home support or after he went into care, it's been important to question things that don't seem right or aren't working, decisions we may not have agreed with, medications being offered, and so on.

We had a situation a couple of years post-diagnosis (thankfully pre-COVID) where Dad required admission into a general hospital to have a pacemaker fitted. This was going to require a stay of 2-3 nights and immediately raised concern for us in terms of his ability to cope with staying in hospital. He couldn't fully understand the background of the procedure, let alone the "rules" about being an inpatient. Initially he was to be placed in a ward with others, and we were told there would be no opportunity for one of us to stay with him in the ward (in a chair overnight, by his bedside). But with a bit of discussion about his situation, and arguing our case, permission was granted not only for him to be admitted into a single room but also for my husband (who is a Nurse Practitioner) and I to take turns staying with him each night in order to manage his confusion about the change of environment and deal with his night-time disturbance. Without question, that arrangement was the best-case scenario for everyone – we didn't need to worry about him from home, he was with someone familiar the whole time, and the hospital avoided having to supervise him one-on-

one over a period of a few days. It was worth putting in a bit of effort to get the best outcome for Dad. And it cost us nothing except a bit of time.

Get your affairs in order

"Confidence comes from being prepared" – John Wooden

None of us can be too prepared for what might be lurking just around the corner. And diagnosing dementia is not like breaking a bone – you don't hear a snap, feel immense pain, have an x-ray, and get confirmation something is broken. It's also not just one thing that happens which makes it immediately obvious to you, and others, that you've got dementia. As you've read, it can sneak up on you, and for us it was a 'slow burn' over a period of five or six years. Mum and Dad already had a Will in place, and I had Enduring Power of Attorney, but it quickly became important for Dad to complete an 'Advanced Health Directive' and 'Statement of Wishes' while he was still able to articulate his thoughts, give consent, and record how he wanted the end of his life to look. **If you haven't done so already, I urge you to have the hard conversations and sort out the big decisions while your loved ones are still able to state their wishes.**

In our case, a local specialist nurse who deals with advance care planning visited us at home, making it relaxed and as easy as possible for both Mum and Dad. It may be different in your area, but I encourage you to take the time to find out what's available to you and your family, and then engage with the process of advance care planning before time is against you. In fact, if there is one thing you get out of this book, I hope it's this message, and that you then spread the word about the importance of future planning to your friends and family. It's something that can help you take back some control (over a disease that can make you feel very out of control), and it can help break down the fear that surrounds not only dementia but end of life in general

– it's about being on the front foot instead of the back one. So, get onto your paperwork, write out your favourite family recipes (that's not something we EVER had to worry about with our no-cooking-Dad!!), make a photo book, or do whatever it is in your family that would be important to have for the future. "Be prepared", as they teach Scouts all over the world.

TAKE-HOME MESSAGE(S) FROM THIS CHAPTER

- In a world where you can be anything, be kind

- Prioritise how you spend your time and who you spend it with, focusing on the people who don't judge you, who don't drain you, whose company you enjoy, and who bring you strength

- In order to find peace, you must accept other people's responses and limitations

- Don't sweat the small stuff – it's often worth a moment of self-reflection to ask yourself, "What's the worst thing that can happen?"

- Stick up for those who may not be able to stick up for themselves

- If you haven't already begun planning for the final years of your life, do it now while you are still able to make your wishes clear to others

CHAPTER EIGHT
HELP AND SUPPORT

You've read about the life lessons we've learned from going through this journey of dementia with Dad, but maybe you're wondering if there is somewhere you can learn more about dementia and where to access help and support.

Yes! In the chapter on Gratitude, I mentioned I undertook an online course. In fact, I completed two courses to learn as much as I could about dementia and what to expect for Dad. I HIGHLY recommend these courses to anyone, and everyone, regardless of whether dementia is part of your family story or not:

- the 'Understanding Dementia MOOC' and

- the 'Preventing Dementia MOOC'

They come out of the University of Tasmania and are offered by the Wicking Dementia Research and Education Centre, global leaders in dementia education.

Both these courses are **100% free**, online, self-paced, and offered at various times throughout the year. The information is easy to follow, the courses are very user-friendly, and you become part of a community of (worldwide) learners as you work your way through the material. I cannot recommend them enough, particularly if you're working in the field or have a friend or family member with dementia, and I have told many others about both courses since I completed them myself. Even if your life has not been touched by dementia, if you're like me and didn't know that maintaining good cardiovascular health, staying connected with others, focusing on the positive relationships in your life, reducing stress, eating well, and exercising might reduce your risk profile for dementia later in life, you might be interested to complete:

- the 'Preventing Dementia MOOC'.

You will learn about the most recent research going on worldwide in this area, and it might just help reduce any fear you may have about dementia.

The drive for this book has been an attempt to reduce negativity, stigma, and fear around dementia, and undertaking these courses certainly helped me in each of those ways. **If you are interested to know more about the courses my husband and I completed, or the others offered by the Wicking Dementia Research and Education Centre, you can check them out at:**

www.utas.edu.au/wicking

In terms of support while Dad lived at home, Mum and I accessed both:

- the National Dementia Helpline (1800 100 500) and

- the Dementia Support Australia helpline (1800 699 799)

Mum was able to pre-book telephone counselling on a couple of occasions via the helpline, which she found reassuring and non-judgemental. There's something particularly "safe" about talking to an unknown person on the phone when you're feeling distressed, in that it provides you with an opportunity to speak openly without the fear of being misinterpreted by those around you.

Wherever you are in the world, I would urge you to seek out whatever in-person or telephone help or support is available in your local area (or nationally), especially if you are feeling alone or like no one else understands what you are experiencing. There may be a carer support group you can join (Mum did for a while), there may be a local Dementia Alliance, and as with everything, there is also a wealth of information online about anything and everything to do with dementia. Knowledge is power. Acquire some knowledge, and you cannot help but feel more empowered.

CONCLUSION

nd so we come to the end of the book, which seems like a good time to elaborate on my reasoning behind the title I chose. I was talking to my good friend Rom one day a few years ago and made the comment that 'Dad had 80 years without dementia'. It was in the context of me reflecting on how I had not felt gutted when Dad received his dementia diagnosis, or at either time he was diagnosed with short-term memory loss before then. This was not because I didn't love my Dad or care about what happened to him – this was because it wasn't the end of his life. He was still around, he was still very much part of the family dynamic, and he was still my Dad. I didn't feel any different toward him, except a bit more protective due to his increased vulnerability. I guess I saw his diagnosis as being the start of the final chapter of his life – a chapter in a very large book that contained all manner of personal achievements, proud moments, challenges, and accomplishments. Yes he was going to end his long and happy life with dementia, but he had eighty years **without** dementia before that, and the diagnosis did not, and would not in the future, define him or the life he had led.

We all have a choice about how we are going to remember our loved ones – just because they may have changed, that change doesn't necessarily dictate how we choose to remember them. Dad is way more than any diagnosis – that is how I have continued to see him, and it's also how I will remember him when he's not here anymore. Exactly the way he was for all those decades when he didn't have dementia.

Even if he is unrecognisable in some of his behaviours and limitations by now, I know for a fact, Dad is very satisfied with the full life he's had. I'm confident he would not want anyone to feel pity or sorrow for him, or see his dementia as representing a shame for things which couldn't happen as previously planned. Remember, he's always been an optimist and never welcomed people lingering around in negativity! In addition to that, I truly believe his soul remains happy – that has been shaped by the positive experiences he's had across more than eight decades, more than six of those being with Mum; they provided a good life to 3 children on a farm, they've done some international travel, he's flown them many places around Australia, they've enjoyed a good social life, and he's done meaningful work in the community and for others. As Mum says;

"Bob is still Bob...sometimes it's hard to remember that when you see him like he is now, but then you think of all the things he's achieved, that we've achieved, that's what you really want to remember".

Before I finish, I would like to very briefly summarise the lessons I have learnt while travelling the dementia path with Dad, those lessons I have described to you throughout the book:

- Caring for someone with dementia at home can be very challenging, and carer burnout is real

- Sometimes you need to trust your intuition, be courageous, and make hard decisions

- We should stop comparing ourselves to others and harbouring the guilt which often results when we do

- It's more satisfying to spend our time living for today, rather than dwelling on the past or worrying excessively for the future

- It's important to seek out (often simple) things to feel grateful for every day

- As long as your intention is to do what you firmly believe to be right, you should minimise regret

- Save your worries for things that really matter – don't sweat the small stuff

- Get your affairs in order, plan ahead for your future

- And remember, there is a 'still a person inside' the diagnosis, and that person still has needs and feelings just like everybody else – continue to include them, show them kindness, give them time, demonstrate empathy, be tolerant, stick up for them when they need you to, keep their best interest at the centre of your intentions, and 'just be there' with whatever needs to happen

As you might imagine, writing this book has been quite an emotional ride, and I have felt the enormity of getting it right quite keenly at times. I have also felt my Dad's presence, as he 'sat by me' urging me on. Although he will not be able to engage with the book in the way he would have previously, I know he'd be super proud of me for conveying the lessons I have learnt (from him) to you, and I know he's pretty chuffed to leave you a parting gift. A legacy from his life. From my own point of view, if this book assists one person or one family, or helps in even a small way to lessen the fear and remove some of the negative stigma around dementia, I will be so much more than happy.

I hope you have enjoyed reading about our journey with dementia as much as I have enjoyed writing it ♥

Lisa
lisa@eightyyearswithoutdementia.com
FB Eighty Years Without Dementia

ACKNOWLEDGEMENTS

First and foremost, I want to acknowledge Mum's contribution to this book. She's been an enthusiastic supporter of this project from the beginning, in fact long before it got off the ground and began taking shape as a written piece of work. But even more importantly than that, she has demonstrated vulnerability, honesty, and openness about the really hard road she's travelled at times and given me her blessing to splash her emotions across the page to a global audience. That takes supreme courage, and I am so humbled she put her trust in me to deliver her very personal words to you the reader. Just as for Dad, I will always love you Mum.

I want to thank my older brothers for being on the end of the phone whenever I've needed them throughout this dementia journey, but also for continuing to support Mum and staying in Dad's life despite the (geographical) distance between us. Special thanks to my eldest brother and sister-in-law for giving the kids a fabulous interstate holiday, which, in turn, delivered me the headspace I needed to write this book.

My very dear friend Rom should take full credit for planting the seed a few years ago that I would write a book one day! Not only did she continue to encourage me all the way, but she also introduced me to Dave, Davina, Rachel, Kez, and the team at Inspirational Book Writers. This book would never have happened without them, and I am eternally grateful they do what they do with so much passion, wisdom, and love.

To the rest of my "support crew" for this project – in particular Susan, Kathy, Heidi, and Kerri-Anne – I say a big thank you for taking an interest in what I was trying to achieve and encouraging me to "just do it"! Good news, I finally did it 😊

And finally…to my beloved hubby, for ALWAYS believing in me, supporting my ideas, and encouraging me to do what I need to do. While I was writing this book, he was halfway around the world on a humanitarian mission with Médecins Sans Frontières, delivering nursing support to the very impoverished nation of Yemen. But while he wasn't present in person, he was on the end of Whatsapp messaging and Google Meet video calls, sending love and support on an ongoing basis. This grounded me, helped me manage the emotional content of the book again and again, and also sent me off to bed at night in a very happy place! As you know very well, I love you beyond Chiron.

NOTES

NOTES